# Survival Communication:

## 15 Proven Tutorials How To Communicate With Your Family When the World Goes Silent

Table of content


Introduction: Language ..........................................................................................3

Chapter 1: Radio Communication.............................................................................6

Communication Hack Number 1: Ham Radio............................................................8

Communication Hack Number 2: C.B. Radio .............................................................9

Communication Hack Number 3: Hand Cranked Radio ...........................................11

Hack Number 4: Packet Radio ................................................................................12

Hack Number 5: Walkie Talkies .............................................................................13

Chapter 2: Phone Technology................................................................................14

Communication hack Number 6: Landline Phones..................................................15

Communication hack Number 7: Satellite Phones ..................................................16

Communication Hack Number 8: Conventional Cell Phones.....................................17

Communication Hack Number 9: Fax Machine .......................................................19

Hack Number 10: Pay Phones................................................................................20

Chapter 3: Unconventional Communication ...........................................................21

Communication Hack Number 11: Morse Code ......................................................21

Communication Hack Number 12: Signal Flares......................................................22

Communication Hack Number 13: Homing Pigeons ................................................23

Communication Hack Number 14: Smoke Signals ...................................................24

Communication Hack Number 15: Message in a Bottle...........................................25

Conclusion: Keep On Trucking ...............................................................................27

## Introduction: Language

Some Urban Preppers are actively looking for a dependable way to communicate in the face of a disaster, but many have not been able to find what they are looking for. Other Preppers don't even give long distance communication a second thought, they figure that when the grid goes, so does any means of reliable communication. But even though communication does take up more resources, establishing contact when the world goes silent is not an impossible feat, and as we delve into the mechanics behind some of these rudimentary efforts, we will show you how.

Because when times become tougher we have to get ready to provide for ourselves what society and the grid may not be able to. And while you are preparing to survive disaster, sooner rather than later you will realize just how important communication is; a need which in many cases ranks every bit as high as food and first aid. In this book I hope to drive that point home.

I myself have read many prepping books that have covered just about every aspect of survival, but everything I have read always tends to be somewhat lacking when it comes to describing an adequate means to communicate during an emergency. This prepping guide intends to finally bridge that gap. Letting you know exactly what you need to do, should your world suddenly go silent.

### *Failure of the Grid and When the World Goes Silent*

The infrastructure of many communities is growing very tenuous and frail after many years of use, and it is only a matter of time before they fail completely. Just think about te scenarios that we might face. The power goes out, the grid fails and our conventional window for speaking to the outside world slams shut, what can we do? Just bow our heads and resign ourselves to our isolated fate.

Absolutely not! Because when the spit hits the fan guys, like any good prepper knows, when one conventional means of anything fails, there are many more unconventional methods that will arise to take their place. Before a crisis erupts, there are several things that you can do to prep your communication potential beforehand.

### Some Basic Communication Prep

First of all you should have what I term an "emergency communication" kit. This kit should have a classic AM/FM battery powered radio with an additional set of extra batteries. You should also have a NOAH radio on hand so you can have access to all of the latest weather alerts.

Another basic communication prep you should pack in your kit is a nifty little device known as a PDA (Personal Digital Assistant) these devices are pretty resourceful, sending out instant text and radio notifications whenever a crisis strikes, providing a lifeline directly to local administrative authorities helping you stay abreast of the situation as it unfolds.

And don't get me wrong with some of the seeming simplicity, because the PDA is not a normal communication device. This baby is special. The main reason why this device is so special is because it is directly linked to the main civil infrastructure in your area, it doesn't piggy back off of other infrastructure, it comes directly from the source. That way, even if 90% of the grid is shut down, you will still be able to get a direct link to the main group of people working hard to save your life.

Along with these standard alert systems you could also inundate yourself with a emergency alert system. What is an emergency alert system? You have probably seen some rather comical commercials in association with this system that involve old people falling down who are unable to get up. (Help! I've fallen and I can't get up!) but as funny as these commercials are and as good of a punch line as they make, the emergency alert system is not a bad idea, and if you really want to prep for when the world goes silent having a good EAS would give you a great head start.

Because once one of these emergency alert systems are set up in your house, as long as the Civil Government is not in complete collapse, EAS will give you immediate access to all fire, police, and emergency services at just the press of a button. This Alert System typically works off of a landline phone, so as old as they are; every prepper should have a landline up as a part of basic communication prep.

We will talk about landline phones more in depth later on in this book. But all you need to know right now, is that as long as the phone line is up, your land line can be a lifeline. So couple this with an ESA and you will have a great means of communication prep at your disposal. These are all great ways to prep when the spit hits the fan and the world begins to go silent.

## Chapter 1: Radio Communication

If the unthinkable happened and the main communication grid of your community was shutdown, what would you do? We are all so used to being linked up to main line communication it would be hard for many of u to adjust. But just because your power goes out, or your main communication grid somehow becomes disrupted there is no need to panic.

There are several ways that we can get around the normal lines of communication in an emergency. The first thing that comes to mind for most people when they think of auxiliary communication tools is that of the old fashioned battery powered radio. These old battery powered AM/FM dialers used to be quite ubiquitous and every house typically had at least one of these devices stashed away somewhere.

In the world of today however, they are rapidly becoming a scarce commodity. Even as recently as 1999, (ironically enough) 99% of all American households were found to have at least 1 radio. That figure has dropped to less than 40% today. A device such as an AM/FM radio has become quite outmoded in the face of live streamed feeds fed to our i-Phones straight off the internet.

And that's just fine as long as the massive infrastructure required to feed that stream in your phone remains unaffected, but this may not always be the case. And if you were going to place your bets on which communication system would most likely remain functioning during a disaster, that simple little radio starts to look like a lot more promising. It is the nature of how radio is broadcast is what lends to its durability, the fact that waves can travel over long distances unimpeded lends credence to this medium's durability.

Cell-phones, as much as we love them, are prone to failure, even if cell phone towers are still available, during a crisis situation, every single person in your area will no doubt be frantically calling everyone they know on their phone and in no time, all of this extra traffic will cause the whole thing to come crashing down. Radio does not have this problem. Unlike cell phones, radios do not need a massive network of receiving stations bouncing signals off of each other.

A typical AM radio signal for example, uses what is known as "amplitude modulation" that takes the amplification of a radio transmission and magnifies them to an incredible extent, with some radio stations sending out broadcasts as high as 500 kW, with a range that can reach the entire planet. This means that if you have even just a tiny little battery powered radio, when dialed to the right AM station you can receive uninterrupted broadcast from anywhere during an emergency.

Emergency broadcasts are typically made at this bandwidth, so it is a great way to stay informed during a chaotic situation. But even more than staying updated by listening to the radio, an even better hack is to be able to communicate *through* the radio, and this can be done anywhere, by anyone, through what is called "ham radio".

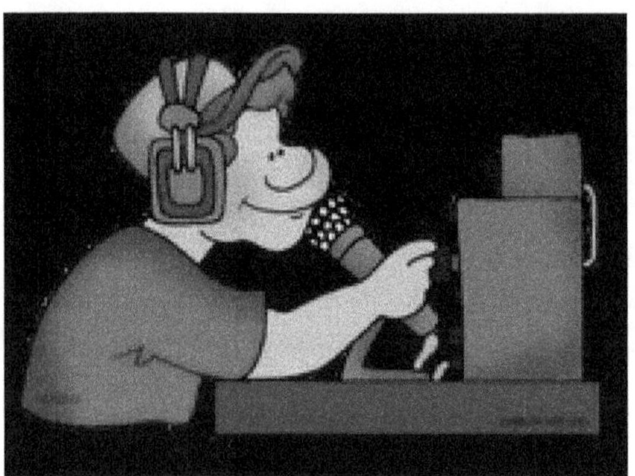

Ham Radios have a huge range when it comes to communication and they can work even in the most limited of infrastructures.  And even if there is a slight disruption in the Ham Radio feed, because of the sheer numbers of operators, ham radio can bounce back rather quickly during times of duress. Ham radio enthusiasts typically arrange their communication nodes into local and regional groups thereby strengthening their signals by doubling up on these locations to expand bandwidth.

And while Ham operators have received the unfair reputation of being, well "Hams" these guys are usually not amateurs at all. And it is not uncommon to find professional teams   of Ham Radio participants working in direct tandem with public safety agencies and law enforcement during times of crisis and emergency.

To set up your Ham Radio; first and foremost you are going to need what is termed a "Rig'. An offshoot of the classic separate receiver and transmitter, the "Rig" is a combination of both of these components, and are placed together in a device that is typically no bigger than a DVD reader.

With the "Rig" in place, you will need to get your hands on a good microphone and a good set of earphones so that you can listen and speak with your transmitter and receiver interchangeably. You will also need a good antenna so that you can pick ham radio signals out of the air. Antennas can range from the size of a pencil piece of wiring, all the way to tree sized, set of steel broadcast towers.

### *Communication Hack Number 2: C.B. Radio*

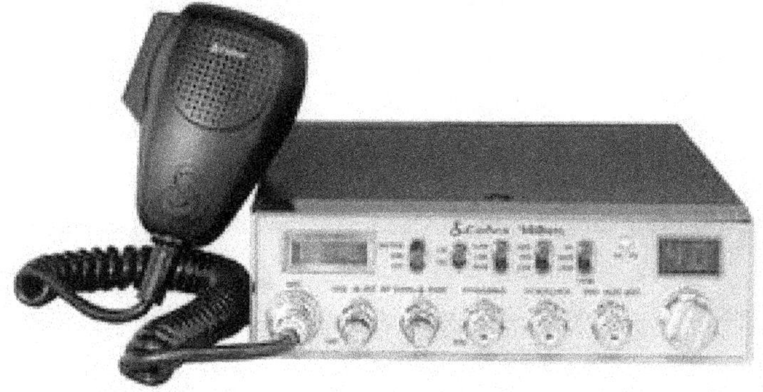

Another famous alternative in radio communication is that of the C.B. Radio. Known around the world as the lifeline of truck drivers, but just as its acronym

(Citizens Band) radio, implies, this medium is perfectly conducive for just about any other citizen around world as well. And since it was introduced as a viable means of communication technology in the early 1960's CB radio has been standard fare fore emergency, police, and transportation agencies worldwide.

CB works on a short wave length of communication over 40 different channels within the 27 MHz band width. Two-way communication with a CB radio works by giving each user a "handle" essentially a place to wait in the queue for their turn to speak. The handle also constitutes the unique nickname by which the user is known by. The handle you choose doesn't have to be anything fancy and quite often a CB handle is something ridiculous.

In fact when I fooled around with the CB circuit I knew a guy who went by the handle of "Big Macho Piece of Crap". Not sure what he was thinking with that one, but the main point is that he created a unique and memorable handle that wouldn't get mixed up with anyone else who was waiting in the queue.

Believe me, I would never forget someone named Big Macho Piece of Crap, it tends to just scream through the airwaves doesn't it? While your creating your name however, one thing to keep in mind is to always keep all of your handles PG Rated because the FCC (Federal Communication Commission) tends to frown upon anything overtly obscene or offensive.

All CB communication has to be done one at a time; this is due to the fact that only one CB station may transmit their communication at any given time since all channels are shared. So although CB communication is an effective means to send a message during a time of duress, it does require a little patience at first to get the word out.

## *Communication Hack Number 3: Hand Cranked Radio*

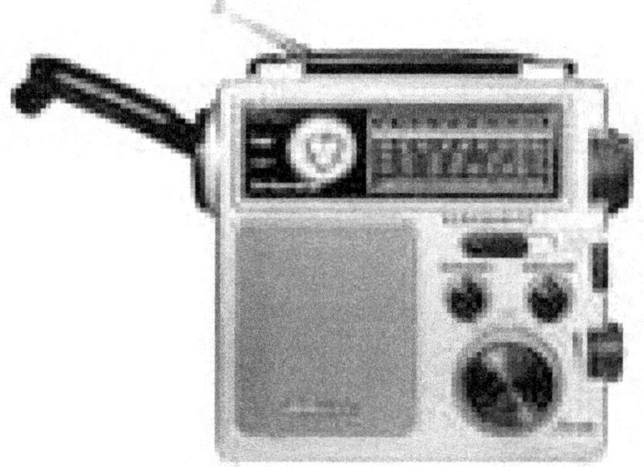

The true definition of a viable "emergency radio" is a failsafe piece of radio equipment that will work when all other standard varieties will not. Much more than a simple battery powered AM/FM that you bought from Wal-Mart; a true "emergency radio" would be able to bring you vital communication for prolonged power outages and even when all of your batteries are dead.

One shining example of this would be the Hand Cranked Radio. Modern hand cranked radios are quite phenomenal, even coming complete with usb ports on the side; with nothing but the power of your forearm you can charge all of your electronic devices. To use a hand crack radio, it's simply, just as you imagined, just grab hold of the lever and start rapidly turning it, the force that you use on the lever is then collected and transferred into energy to charge up the device.

# Hack Number 4: Packet Radio

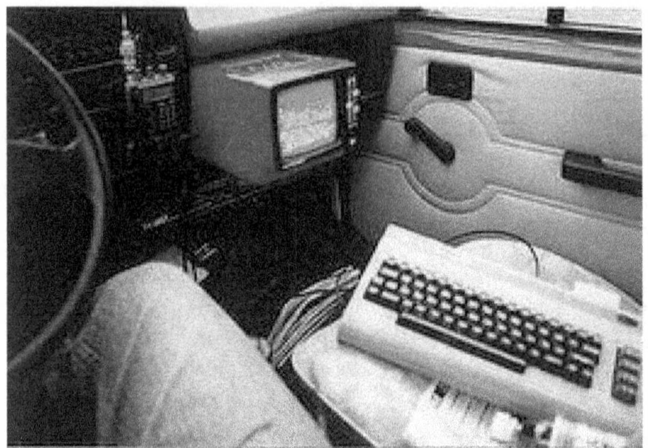

Working on an early version of the modern text message, packet radio can transmit up to 256 characters over the radio waves. Typically this is achieved through a computer working as an interface between the keyboard and the radio's receiver. When text is received through Packet Radio it will either appear on the screen or as a print out. Packet Radio is a great unsung hero of survival communication.

## *Hack Number 5: Walkie Talkies*

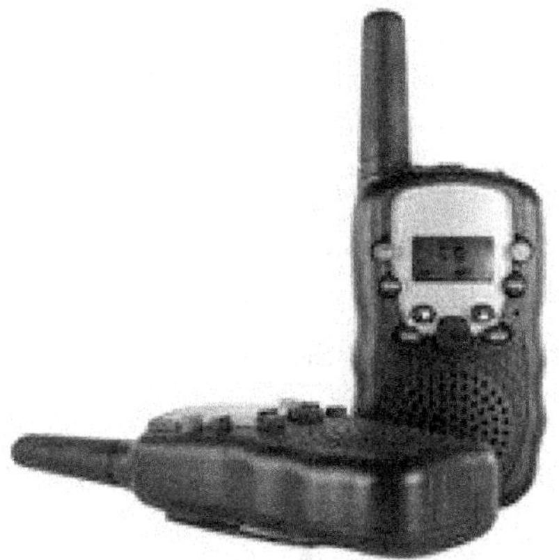

As a kid I used to love playing with these, me and my friends had a pair and we would spend endless hours pretending to be on secret missions as we radioed each other over our walkie talkies. A walkie talkie is basically a mobile radio receiver. It usually comes with multiple channels that it can be set to for receipt of any broadcast.

In order to transmit your own communication you press a button on the side of the device which then switches the walkie talkie into a sending device transmitting your speech to the other recipients. This two way communication is a bit slower since it can only be done one at a time, but if you have nothing else to communicate with, it could serve you well if the rest of the world ever does go silent.

## Chapter 2: Phone Technology

Although we have already outlined the frailty of certain telephone infrastructure, if used wisely you still could use this technology as an emergency window into the outside world. Telephones have had a long evolution with the very first incarnation of this technology coming to us in the form of the Telegraph all the way back in 1816.

The Telegraph of course would later morph into the telephone which would then eventually springboard us into the communication technology explosion of today with cell phones, satellite phones, and all the rest. Phone technology has revolutionized the world that we live in more than the creators of the Telegraph and the original Telephone could have ever imagined.

The phone began as a mostly civil and military application with governments wishing to convey logistics and raw data over the telegraph wires. The telegraph's successor the telephone then quickly found its way in every family's home, and now expand this evolutionary rate of growth further, every single member of a family has their own personal phone in their pocket.

We are now dependent on phone technology more than ever, and when an emergency hits, the overwhelmed grid bears a stark testament to that fact. Having that said, with so much good and also so much that could go wrong with these devices, we are going to take a nice and sober look at just what value can be pulled from the world of phone technology when the world goes silent.

## <u>*Communication hack Number 6: Landline Phones*</u>

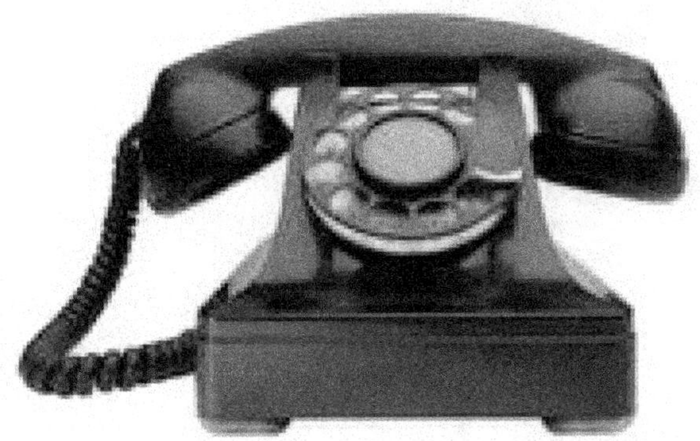

Yes they still exist. Even though they are becoming a rare household item for many, the infrastructure never left us, the miles of phone lines are still in place and the landline phone is still an option. But when push comes to shove, just how reliable are they? Well a lot of that depends on the location and environmental factors that are involved. Physical landlines are extremely susceptible to strong winds that can bring the lines down. Phone lines can also be shorted out by electrical surges.

But as long as the physical line lasts, the landline phone is a great way to contact the outside world. As mentioned before, high volume cell phone use during emergencies tend to jam the line and cause networks to crash, but this kind of logjam does not occur on landline phones. So as long as these physical landline cables exist they really could help us out in an emergency.


### _Communication hack Number 7: Satellite Phones_

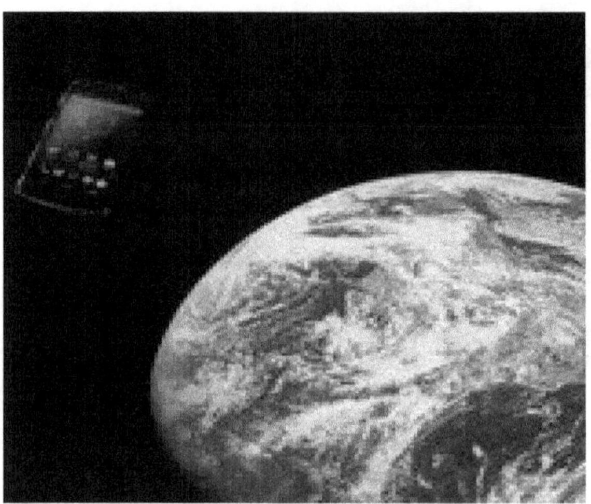

In most emergencies Satellite Phones should remain reliable. This resilience does come with a cost however, because most Satellite Phones are fairly expensive. You have to pay a good chunk of change for the phone itself and then on top of that you will also have to pay high priced fees in order to start up your service. I hate to break it to you, but if you thought that just because a signal is constantly being beamed down by a satellite it is free, this is sadly not the case.


But if you can afford it, these Satellite phones could prove to be an invaluable lifeline. And unless another country launches a satellite killing missile or space aliens decide to fry the crap out of your Sat (you never know right?), without one of these extraordinarily rare hypothetical's occurring, there is a 99.9% chance that your satellite feed will remain uninterrupted during a crisis. This means that the entire infrastructure on the ground could be wiped out, but as long as that happy little satellite is orbiting the planet from space, you will always have a way to talk, even if the rest of the world goes silent.

### *Communication Hack Number 8: Conventional Cell Phones*

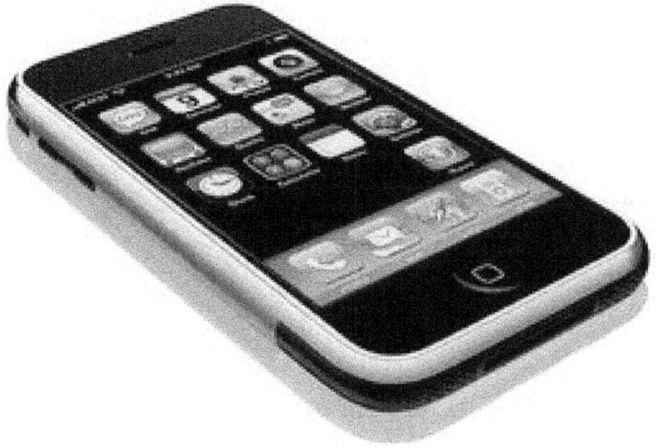

I know that we have already pointed out all the glaring vulnerabilities of this device, but since practically all of us have a cell phone on us at all times, we would be remiss if we did not highlight the best ways to use this technology in an emergency. For starters, you have to keep in mind that a cell phone can be used for much more than making phone calls.

Most of us have smart phones with hundreds of apps attached to them, and among all of these applications, you could find many good hacks around the conventional mode of speaking through them. First of all, if you find that you can not place a call during an emergency because of problems keeping a signal or overloaded networks, instead of calling, try sending out a simple text message instead.

This may seem a bit obvious to some, but the reality is, a text message takes less bandwidth than a regular phone call does, so in a disaster when resource are strained, your text messages will have a much better chance of getting through due to this narrower bandwidth allotment. This is why text would be preferable to a standard phone call.

Most emergency number such as 911 accept text messages now too, so if you truly need to get some sort of emergency aid, there is no shame in texting your request, a simple text and you will have emergency responders right on the scene. Along with text, you may also want to try other data options on your phone such as sending a simple e-mail or even seeing if you can update your friends and family of your status through mobile social media such as face book and twitter.

## Communication Hack Number 9: Fax Machine

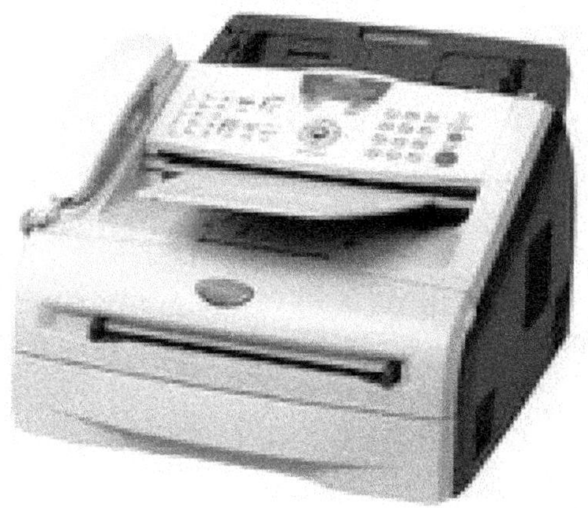

The old standard Fax Machine hooked up to your phone line is probably the last piece of communication equipment that you would think to use in an emergency. But if you were left with no other recourse, you could commandeer your fax and use it almost like you would your e-mail. Because if you had nothing else but a fax line, a pen, and a piece of paper, you could simply write up emergency memo's and fax them off to whoever you think might be listening when the world goes silent.

_Hack Number 10: Pay Phones_
=====

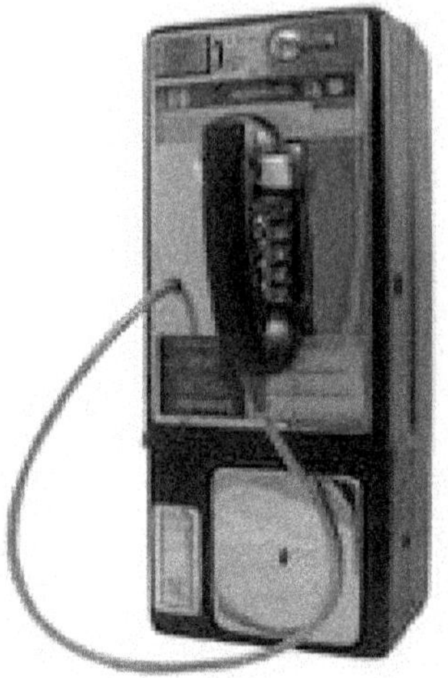

Most people probably think that this kind of phone has kicked the bucket for good, but this is not the case. There are still public pay phones located in just about any region you could think of. And if you are having trouble finding the ones near you, there are whole sites and apps dedicated to making that search easier. So if your cell signal is shot to hell but you have just enough data to use some apps on your smart phone, you could use them to locate that old fashioned public payphone just around the corner. These are all just a few phone hacks to cut through the silence.

## Chapter 3: Unconventional Communication

The concept of communication is so broad and diverse; it is not limited to the standard bearing technologies. And there are several other hacks that can get you around them. Whether it is through light displays, smoke signals, or even a message in a bottle, where there is a will; there is communication.

Just because standard technology and the grid has failed you doesn't mean that you can not use a little bit of ingenuity and begin work on your very own means of communication. So that no matter how quiet the world gets, if you try hard enough you will be able to get your message across. Having that said, let us check out these great unconventional forms of communication just in case the Spit Hits The Fan and the whole world should go silent around us.

### *Communication Hack Number 11: Morse Code*

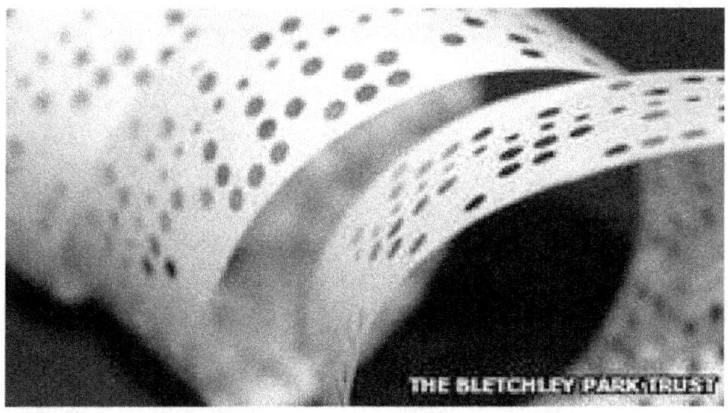

Morse code is a classic mode of communication which was developed to transmit messages through a precise series of clicks, lights, or tones. This can be accomplished through either flashing a light, emitting a specific tone from electronic equipment or even by beating its precise rhythm with a drum.

This special language is understood all over the world. It is so basic and so automatic that even the guys at SETI (Search for Extra Terrestrial Intelligence) have proposed to use it in attempts at contacting alien civilizations! The accepted language of Morse Code is able to encapsulate all of the written alphabet and numerals and represent them with a series of dots and dashes which are the written equivalent of short and long bursts of sound/lights as they are interpreted by the recipient.

### _Communication Hack Number 12: Signal Flares_

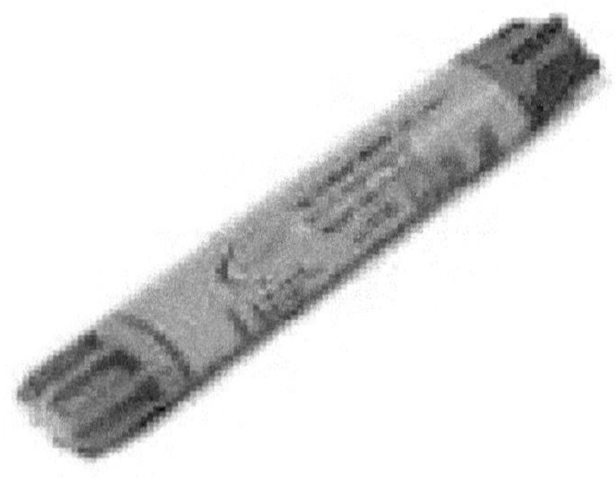

Flares are great in an emergency and are not to be discounted when it comes to communicating distress to emergency response personnel. Flares send up powerful flashes of light that can attract attention by air, land and sea. If you don't have any other means of sending out a flare, the standard means of signaling would require you to start three fires that form a triangle and are large enough to be seen from the air.

This flaming triangle is part of an international standard in emergency communication and will immediately notify any rescue teams of your call for help. The best and easiest way to get the attention of first responders however would be to use a good flare gun. Every prepper should have a flare gun in their emergency arsenal, just in case they need to notify someone on the outside in a hurry.

## *Communication Hack Number 13: Homing Pigeons*

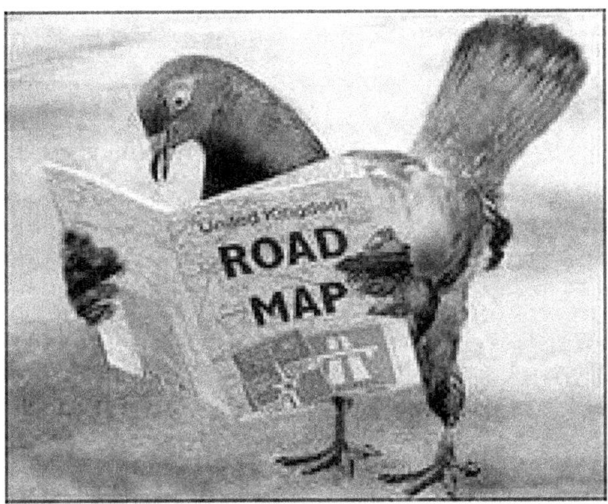


Birds such as Pigeons have been used for thousands of years to relay messages of long distances. They are still used by various civil and military operations around the globe. The premise of this communication is simple. You take a bird who is used to calling a certain locale home, and then distribute it to far away locations.

When the far away location would like to communicate and write back to the place of origin, he simply attaches messages to the bird and then lets it go. The bird will then automatically fly back home with the messages attached. This method could be used in an emergency by getting birds from an official emergency location and then releasing them if and when you may need assistance. Sending out your call for help attached to the tiny little feet of a bird.

### ***Communication Hack Number 14: Smoke Signals***

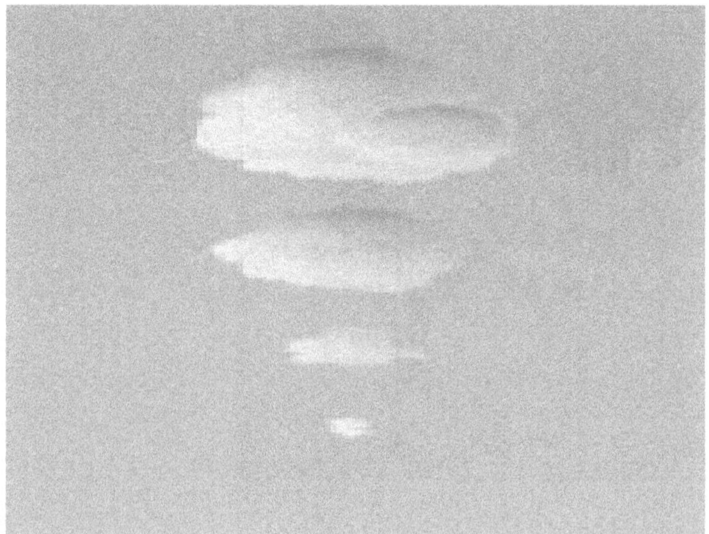

Just like flares, smoke signals work upon the visual senses to solicit aid. Smoke signals have been used for thousands of years, and most notably Native Americans used them to signal to each other all over the American West. The premise of smoke signals is simplistic but effective; similar to Morse code, the smoke is manipulated in order to convey specific messages. Traditionally a rug or some other flat material is used to cover the smoke and intermittently changing the velocity and pathway of the smoke, thereby creating a means of communication.

## *Communication Hack Number 15: Message in a Bottle*

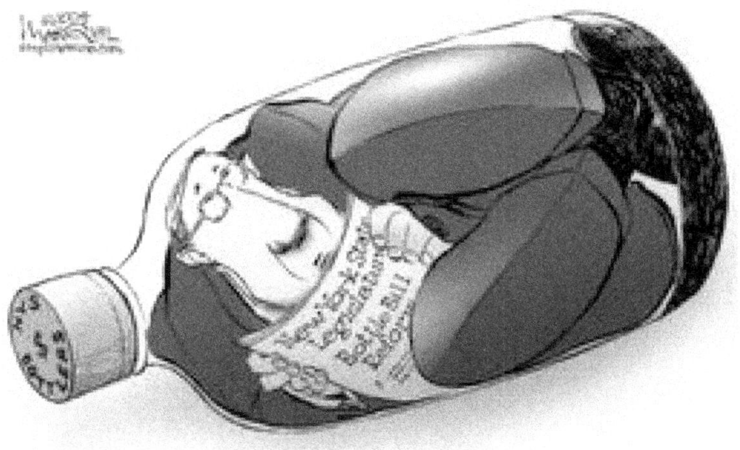

This is an unconventional means of communication that could be used if you live near a large body of water. Admittedly this one would most likely be used as a last ditch effort if all other communication means had failed. But if you find yourself stranded somewhere and you put a clear and concise message with the exact coordinates of your location included, you may just get saved. U.S. navy and other official personnel will responded to an S.O.S.—even delivered via a message in a bottle.

## Conclusion: Keep On Trucking

When most guys here that line they probably start shaking in fear because they think that their girlfriend is about to break up with them! But the phrase carries much more meaning to us when we are thinking of ways to survive in a world gone silent. We all need communication. Communication is almost written into the very DNA of what it means to be a human being.

Scientists say that the first human dialogue was established as long as 500,000 years ago. Pretty mind blowing when you think about it, because for about half a million years human beings have not stopped talking. Quite a tradition and one that civilization should carry on with. We are lost if we can not communicate with each other. This is a point that this book has sought to hammer home while introducing tried and true methods to break through the static, no matter what the emergency.

I first became enamored with off the grid communication when my older brother introduced me to CB radio as a kid. The CB rig we had was actually inherited from my uncle Rocky who was a truck driver. When we started using this thing it was in the early 1990's before there was an internet or cell phones or any real means of communication besides the landline phone.

I remember how exhilarating it was on the CB radio to just tune into a frequency and then suddenly be able to join in on a conversation with random people from all over the place. It was as if a whole new world was opened up to us just by using a cheap piece of radio equipment.

It was this first foray into CB Radio that got me hooked on survival communication and now that I am a little older and I have experienced all of the other aspects of modern communication, I can still appreciate that old CB Radio and the promise of unhindered dialogue that it brings. So even if the world ever goes silent I'll still have my handle and be able to keep right on trucking.

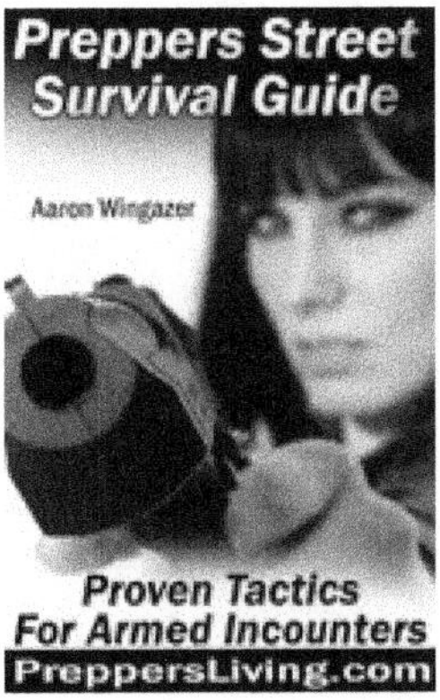

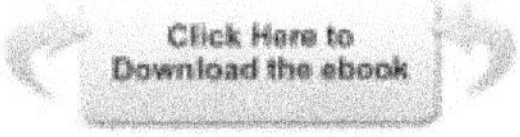

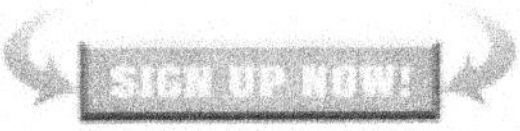

OR Go to this URL
**http://zbit.ly/1WBb1Ek**

www.ingramcontent.com/pod-product-compliance
Lightning Source LLC
Chambersburg PA
CBHW061928270726
48660CB00003BA/1103